DIVINE HEALTH
AFFIRMATIONS
AGAINST
EYE PROBLEMS

...A Therapy that works...

BY
IHEKE WILLIAMS

Unless otherwise indicated, all scripture quotations are taken from the King James Version of the Bible A key for other Bible versions used;

NKJV	New King James Version
AMP	The Amplified Bible
TANT	The New Amplified Bible
TLB -	The Living Bible
CEV -	Contemporary English Version
NASB	New American Standard Version
GW -	God's Word version
ESV -	English Standard Version
NET -	New English Translation
ISV -	International Standard Version
NIV -	New International Version
MSG -	The Message Translation

DEDICATION

This Book is dedicated to Almighty God and
to everyone in the world.

TABLE OF CONTENT

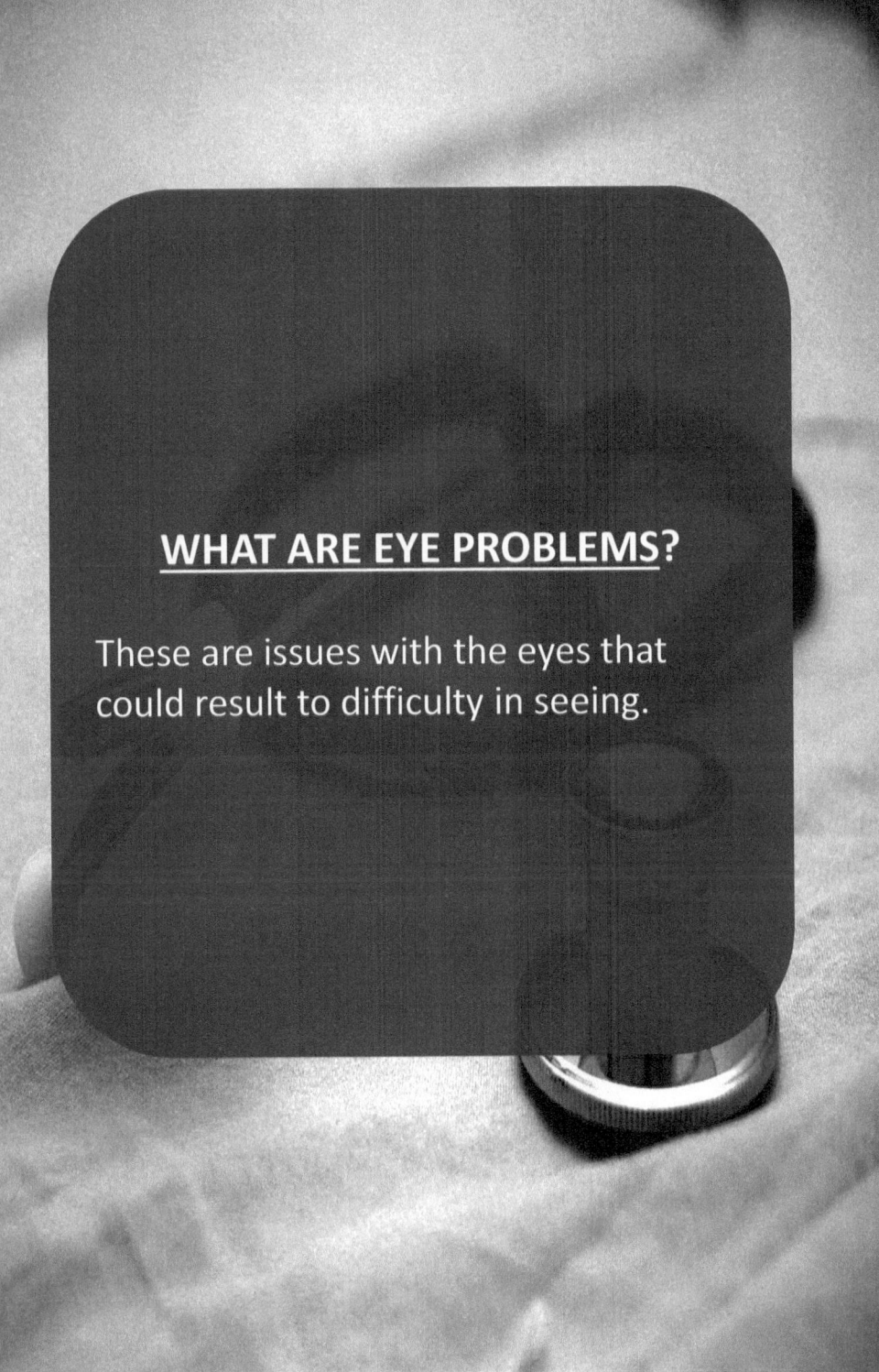

WHAT ARE EYE PROBLEMS?

These are issues with the eyes that could result to difficulty in seeing.

WHAT IS GOD'S SOLUTION

"...By His wounds ye have been healed.."
1 Peter 2:24

JESUS has already healed you over 2000 years ago.

Your eye sight is Active and strong FOREVER because of the wound Jesus suffered on the cross for your sake.

You have NO business with blindness or bad eye sight.

For the next 31 days, you will affirm this blessing in your life that your sight will be perfect FOREVER!

<u>INSTRUCTION 1</u>

That if thou shalt confess with thy mouth the Lord Jesus, and shalt believe in thine heart that God hath raised him from the dead, thou shalt be saved. – Romans 10:9

There has to be a connection with what you say and what you have in your heart. We believe with our heart, this is the reason you have to meditate on the gospel with your heart, believe it and then affirm it with your mouth.

For the affirmations to be effective, you will have to meditate on the scripture (1Peter 2:24) for 5 minutes, in your heart, and then affirm it with your mouth.

INSTRUCTION 2

"For our light affliction, which is but for a moment, worketh for us a far more exceeding and eternal weight of glory;

While we look not at the things which are seen, but at the things which are not seen: for the things which are seen are temporal; but the things which are not seen are eternal. –
2 Corinthians 4:17-18

Don't look at the mirror or yourself during the duration of the affirmation. It affects the word in your heart when you keep seeing the effects of the disease on your body.

Do not touch your eyes.

Don't talk about eyes problems. Only affirm the Blessings you have received from the Lord Jesus Christ on the cross in 1 Peter 2:24

Follow these instructions and your affirmations will be effective.

DAY 1
AFFIRMATION

Meditate on 1 Peter 2:24B in your heart for 5 minutes

"..By His stripes ye have been healed"

Now say the following words to yourself

"I HAVE BEEN HEALED THEREFORE, I AFFIRM THAT MY EYE-SIGHT IS ACTIVE AND PERFECT FOREVER!"

DAY 2
AFFIRMATION

Meditate on 1 Peter 2:24B in your heart for 5 minutes

"..By His stripes ye have been healed"

Now say the following words to yourself

"I HAVE BEEN HEALED THEREFORE, I AFFIRM THAT MY EYE - SIGHT IS ACTIVE AND STRONG FOREVER !"

DAY 3
AFFIRMATION

Meditate on 1 Peter 2:24B in your heart for 5 minutes

"..By His stripes ye have been healed"

Now say the following words to yourself

"I HAVE BEEN HEALED THEREFORE, I AFFIRM THAT MY EYE - SIGHT IS ACTIVE AND STRONG FOREVER!"

DAY 4
AFFIRMATION

Meditate on 1 Peter 2:24B in your heart for 5 minutes

"..By His stripes ye have been healed"

Now say the following words to yourself

"I HAVE BEEN HEALED THEREFORE, I AFFIRM THAT MY EYE - SIGHT IS ACTIVE AND PERFECT FOREVER!"

DAY 5
AFFIRMATION

Meditate on 1 Peter 2:24B in your heart for 5 minutes

"..By His stripes ye have been healed"

Now say the following words to yourself

"I HAVE BEEN HEALED THEREFORE, I AFFIRM THAT MY EYE - SIGHT IS ACTIVE AND STRONG FOREVER!"

DAY 6
AFFIRMATION

Meditate on 1 Peter 2:24B in your heart for 5 minutes

"..By His stripes ye have been healed"

Now say the following words to yourself

"I HAVE BEEN HEALED THEREFORE, I AFFIRM THAT MY EYE - SIGHT IS ACTIVE AND PERFECT FOREVER !"

DAY 7
AFFIRMATION

Meditate on 1 Peter 2:24B in your heart for 5 minutes

"..By His stripes ye have been healed"

Now say the following words to yourself

"I HAVE BEEN HEALED THEREFORE, I AFFIRM THAT MY EYE - SIGHT IS ACTIVE AND STRONG FOREVER!"

DAY 8
AFFIRMATION

Meditate on 1 Peter 2:24B in your heart for 5 minutes

"..By His stripes ye have been healed"

Now say the following words to yourself

"I HAVE BEEN HEALED THEREFORE, I AFFIRM THAT MY EYE - SIGHT IS ACTIVE AND PERFECT FOREVER !"

DAY 9
AFFIRMATION

Meditate on 1 Peter 2:24B in your heart for 5 minutes

"..By His stripes ye have been healed"

Now say the following words to yourself

"I HAVE BEEN HEALED THEREFORE, I AFFIRM THAT MY EYE - SIGHT IS ACTIVE AND STRONG FOREVER!"

DAY 10
AFFIRMATION

Meditate on 1 Peter 2:24B in your heart for 5 minutes

"..By His stripes ye have been healed"

Now say the following words to yourself

"I HAVE BEEN HEALED THEREFORE, I AFFIRM THAT MY EYE - SIGHT IS ACTIVE AND PERFECT FOREVER!"

DAY 11
AFFIRMATION

Meditate on 1 Peter 2:24B in your heart for 5 minutes

"..By His stripes ye have been healed"

Now say the following words to yourself

"I HAVE BEEN HEALED THEREFORE, I AFFIRM THAT MY EYE - SIGHT IS ACTIVE AND STRONG FOREVER !"

DAY 12
AFFIRMATION

Meditate on 1 Peter 2:24B in your heart for 5 minutes

"..By His stripes ye have been healed"

Now say the following words to yourself

"I HAVE BEEN HEALED THEREFORE, I AFFIRM THAT MY EYE - SIGHT IS ACTIVE AND PERFECT FOREVER !"

DAY 13
AFFIRMATION

Meditate on 1 Peter 2:24B in your heart for 5 minutes

"..By His stripes ye have been healed"

Now say the following words to yourself

"I HAVE BEEN HEALED THEREFORE, I AFFIRM THAT MY EYE - SIGHT IS ACTIVE AND STRONG FOREVER!"

DAY 14
AFFIRMATION

Meditate on 1 Peter 2:24B in
your heart for 5 minutes

" ..By His stripes ye have been
healed"

Now say the following words to
yourself

"I HAVE BEEN HEALED THEREFORE, I AFFIRM THAT MY EYE - SIGHT IS ACTIVE AND PERFECT FOREVER !"

DAY 15
AFFIRMATION

Meditate on 1 Peter 2:24B in your heart for 5 minutes

"..By His stripes ye have been healed"

Now say the following words to yourself

"I HAVE BEEN HEALED THEREFORE, I AFFIRM THAT MY EYE - SIGHT IS ACTIVE AND STRONG FOREVER!"

DAY 16
AFFIRMATION

Meditate on 1 Peter 2:24B in your heart for 5 minutes

"..By His stripes ye have been healed"

Now say the following words to yourself

"I HAVE BEEN HEALED THEREFORE, I AFFIRM THAT MY EYE - SIGHT IS ACTIVE AND PERFECT FOREVER!"

DAY 17
AFFIRMATION

Meditate on 1 Peter 2:24B
in your heart for 5 minutes
"..By His stripes ye have
been healed"

Now say the following words
to yourself

"I HAVE BEEN HEALED THEREFORE, I AFFIRM THAT MY EYE - SIGHT IS ACTIVE AND STRONG FOREVER!"

DAY 18
AFFIRMATION

Meditate on 1 Peter 2:24B in your heart for 5 minutes

"..By His stripes ye have been healed"

Now say the following words to yourself

"I HAVE BEEN HEALED THEREFORE, I AFFIRM THAT MY EYE - SIGHT IS ACTIVE AND PERFECT FOREVER!"

DAY 19
AFFIRMATION

Meditate on 1 Peter 2:24B in your heart for 5 minutes

"..By His stripes ye have been healed"

Now say the following words to yourself

"I HAVE BEEN HEALED THEREFORE, I AFFIRM THAT MY EYE - SIGHT IS ACTIVE AND STRONG FOREVER !"

DAY 20
AFFIRMATION

Meditate on 1 Peter 2:24B in your heart for 5 minutes

"..By His stripes ye have been healed"

Now say the following words to yourself

"I HAVE BEEN HEALED THEREFORE, I AFFIRM THAT MY EYE - SIGHT IS ACTIVE AND PERFECT FOREVER!"

DAY 21
AFFIRMATION

Meditate on 1 Peter 2:24B in your heart for 5 minutes

"..By His stripes ye have been healed"

Now say the following words to yourself

"I HAVE BEEN HEALED THEREFORE, I AFFIRM THAT MY EYE - SIGHT IS ACTIVE AND STRONG FOREVER

DAY 22
AFFIRMATION

Meditate on 1 Peter 2:24B in your heart for 5 minutes

"..By His stripes ye have been healed"

Now say the following words to yourself

"I HAVE BEEN HEALED THEREFORE, I AFFIRM THAT MY EYE - SIGHT IS ACTIVE AND PERFECT FOREVER!"

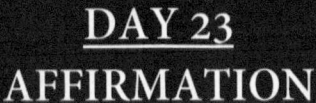

DAY 23
AFFIRMATION

Meditate on 1 Peter 2:24B
in your heart for 5 minutes

"..By His stripes ye have
been healed.."

Now say the following words
to yourself

"I HAVE BEEN HEALED THEREFORE, I AFFIRM THAT MY EYE - SIGHT IS ACTIVE AND STRONG FOREVER!"

DAY 24
AFFIRMATION

Meditate on 1 Peter 2:24B in your heart for 5 minutes

"..By His stripes ye have been healed.."

Now say the following words to yourself

"I HAVE BEEN HEALED THEREFORE, I AFFIRM THAT MY EYE - SIGHT IS ACTIVE AND PERFECT FOREVER!"

DAY 25
AFFIRMATION

Meditate on 1 Peter 2:24B in your heart for 5 minutes

"..By His stripes ye have been healed.."

Now say the following words to yourself

"I HAVE BEEN HEALED THEREFORE, I AFFIRM THAT MY EYE - SIGHT IS ACTIVE AND STRONG FOREVER!"

DAY 26
AFFIRMATION

Meditate on 1 Peter 2:24B in your heart for 5 minutes
"..By His stripes ye have been healed.."

Now say the following words to yourself

"I HAVE BEEN HEALED THEREFORE, I AFFIRM THAT MY EYE - SIGHT IS ACTIVE AND PERFECT FOREVER!"

DAY 27
AFFIRMATION

Meditate on 1 Peter 2:24B in your heart for 5 minutes

"..By His stripes ye have been healed.."

Now say the following words to yourself

"I HAVE BEEN HEALED THEREFORE, I AFFIRM THAT MY EYE - SIGHT IS ACTIVE AND STRONG FOREVER!"

DAY 28
AFFIRMATION

Meditate on 1 Peter 2:24B
in your heart for 5 minutes

"..By His stripes ye have
been healed"

Now say the following words to
yourself

"I HAVE BEEN HEALED THEREFORE, I AFFIRM THAT MY EYE - SIGHT IS ACTIVE AND PERFECT FOREVER!"

DAY 29
AFFIRMATION

Meditate on 1 Peter 2:24B in
your heart for 5 minutes

"..By His stripes ye have
been healed"

Now say the following words to
yourself

"I HAVE BEEN HEALED THEREFORE, I AFFIRM THAT MY EYE - SIGHT IS ACTIVE AND STRONG FOREVER !"

DAY 30
AFFIRMATION

Meditate on 1 Peter 2:24B in your heart for 5 minutes

"..By His stripes ye have been healed"

Now say the following words to yourself

"I HAVE BEEN HEALED THEREFORE, I AFFIRM THAT MY EYE - SIGHT IS ACTIVE AND STRONG FOREVER!"

DAY 31
AFFIRMATION

Meditate on 1 Peter 2:24B in
your heart for 5 minutes

"..By His stripes ye have been
healed"

Now say the following words to
yourself

"I HAVE BEEN HEALED THEREFORE, I AFFIRM THAT MY EYE - SIGHT IS ACTIVE AND STRONG FOREVER!"

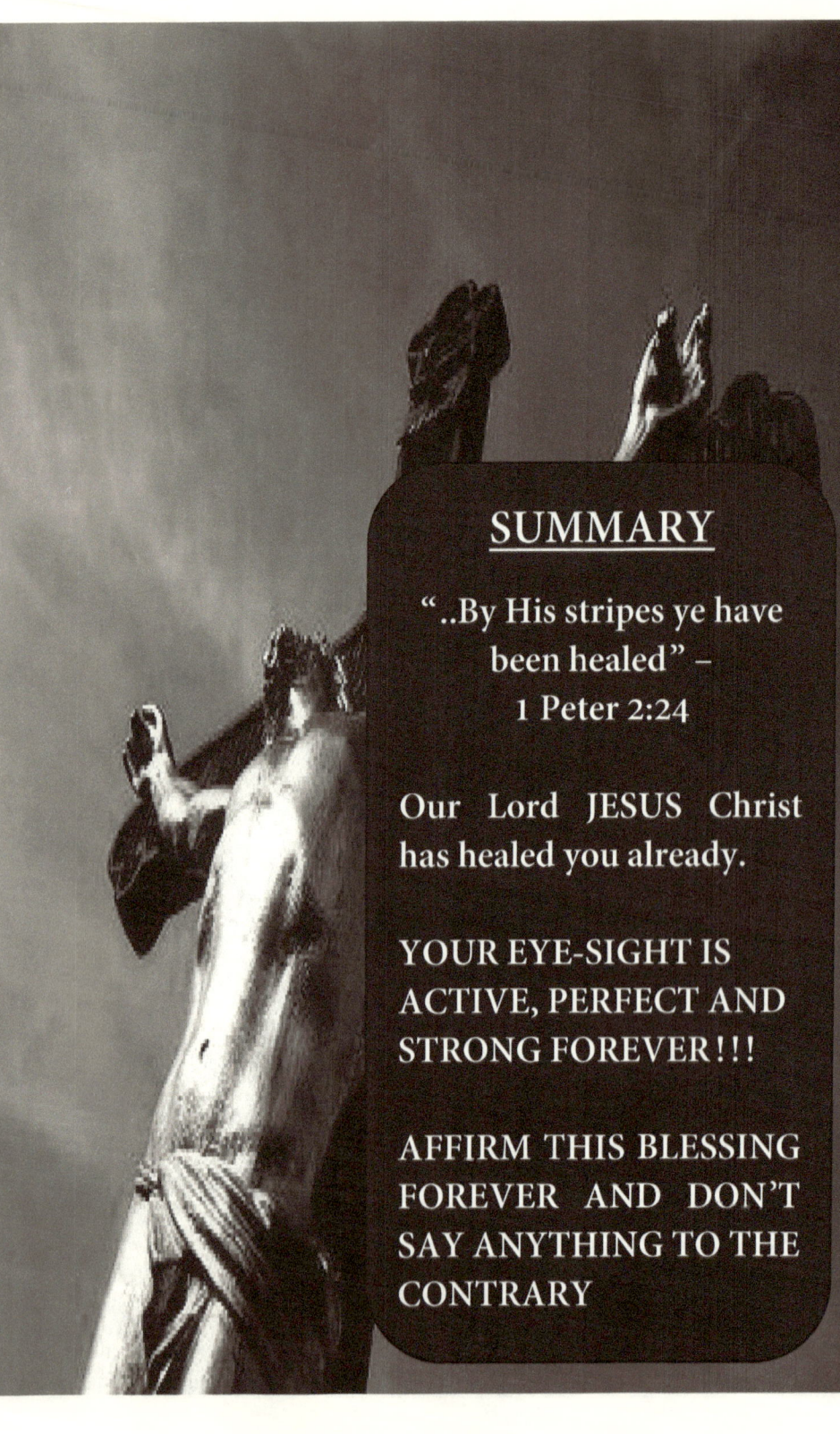

SUMMARY

"..By His stripes ye have been healed" –
1 Peter 2:24

Our Lord JESUS Christ has healed you already.

YOUR EYE-SIGHT IS ACTIVE, PERFECT AND STRONG FOREVER!!!

AFFIRM THIS BLESSING FOREVER AND DON'T SAY ANYTHING TO THE CONTRARY

PRAYER FOR SALVATION

We believe that you have been blessed and that you want to receive eternal life that God has made available to everyone who believes in his love and his grace which He expressed lavishly through His Son Jesus Christ.

"For God so loved the world, that He gave his only begotten Son, that whosoever <u>believeth</u> in him should not perish, but <u>have everlasting life.</u>" - John 3:16

Say this prayer to God and believe it with your heart

"Father, I believe that you gave me your only Son to die for my sin. I believe you raised Him from the dead. I declare that your son, Jesus Christ is the Lord of my life. I receive eternal life and I receive the Holy Spirit. I am saved forever.in Jesus name. I am so Happy that today and forever, I am your child. Amen ".

Congratulations, you are now a child of God Halleluyah!! – John 1:12

OTHER INFORMATION

Please share your testimonies via the following handles;

ihekewilliams@gmail.com
+2348061530541

Other Books written by the author includes

Dad, Pray for your Daughter
Mum, Pray for your Daughter
Mum, pray for your Son
Don't stop the flow of the Blessing
Daddy's Prayers
Mummy's Prayers
Divine Health Affirmations Against Arthritis
Divine Health Affirmations Against HIV
Divine Health Affirmations Series

ABOUT THE AUTHOR

Iheke Williams is a firm follower and disciple of the Lord Jesus Christ. He is a passionate minister of the grace of our Lord and savior Jesus Christ and has brought the reality of the divine life of Christ into the lives of so many.

Iheke Williams has a calling to communicate the gospel of Christ with simplicity and to show the world how to activate the eternal life of God that is in us already which includes Divine health, Divine righteousness, Divine security and Divine prosperity.

As you read this book and other books written by Iheke Williams you will literally begin to function and manifest the life of God that is already inside you to the glory of God the Father who is the author of all grace and mercy. Amen!

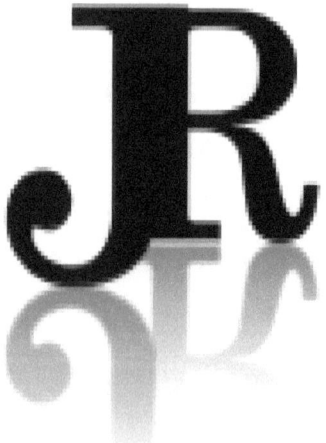

www.ingramcontent.com/pod-product-compliance
Lightning Source LLC
Chambersburg PA
CBHW031334290526
45784CB00014B/2701